Super Simple Comfort Food Recipe Collection for Everybody

The essential tasty and cheap comfort food recipes for everyday meal

Laura Evans

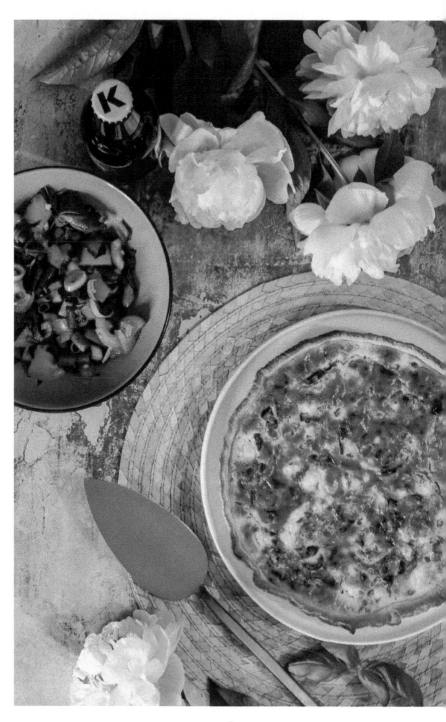

professional advice. The content within this book has been derived from various sources. Please consult a licensed professional before attempting any techniques outlined in this book.

By reading this document, the reader agrees that under no circumstances is the author responsible for any losses, direct or indirect, which are incurred as a result of the use of information contained within this document, including, but not limited to, — errors, omissions, or inaccuracies.

Table of Contents

Walnut Carrot Cake

Preparation time: 10 minutes | Cooking Time: 40 minutes | Servings: 8

Ingredients:

3 eggs

1 tsp baking powder

2/3 cup swerve

1 cup almond flour

3/4 cup walnuts, chopped

1 cup carrot, shredded

1/2 cup heavy cream

1/4 cup coconut oil

1 tsp apple pie spice

Directions:

Spray a baking dish with cooking spray and set it aside.

Add all ingredients into the large bowl and mix with a hand mixer until well combined.

Pour batter into the baking dish and cover the dish with foil.

Pour 2 cups of water into the Pressure Pot then place a trivet in the pot.

Place cake dish on top of the trivet.

Seal pot with lid and cook on manual high pressure for 40 minutes.

Once done then allow to release pressure naturally for 10 minutes then release using the quick-release method. Open the lid.

Carefully remove the dish from the pot and let it cool.

Slice and serve.

Nutrition:

Calories 208, Fat 19.9g, Carbohydrates 24.1g, Sugar 21.1g, Protein 5.9g, Cholesterol 72mg.

Cinnamon Plums

Preparation time: 25 minutes | Cooking Time: 40 minutes | Servings: 4

Ingredients:

4 plums; halved

3 tbsp. Swerve

4 tbsp. Butter; melted

2 tsp. Cinnamon powder

Directions:

In a pan that fits your air fryer, mix the plums with the rest of the ingredients, toss, put the pan in the air fryer and cook at 300°f for 20 minutes

Divide into cups and serve cold.

Nutrition:

Calories 162, Fat 3g, Fiber 2g, Carbs 4g, Protein 5g.

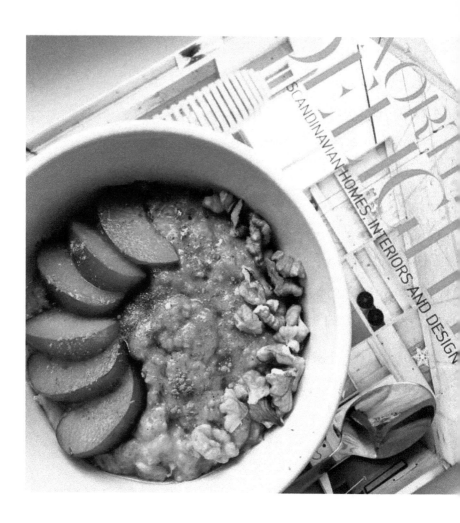

Strawberry Cake

Preparation time: 45 minutes | Cooking Time: 40 minutes | Servings: 6

Ingredients:

1 lb. Strawberries; chopped.

1 egg, whisked

1 cup almond flour

¼ cup swerve

1 cup cream cheese, soft

3 tbsp. Coconut oil; melted

1 tbsp. Lime juice

1 tsp. Vanilla extract

2 tsp. Baking powder

Directions:

Take a bowl and mix all the ingredients, stir well, and pour this into a cake pan lined with parchment paper.

Put the pan in the air fryer, cook at 350°f for 35 minutes, cool down, slice, and serve

Nutrition:

Calories 200, Fat 6g, Fiber 2g, Carbs 4g, Protein 6g.

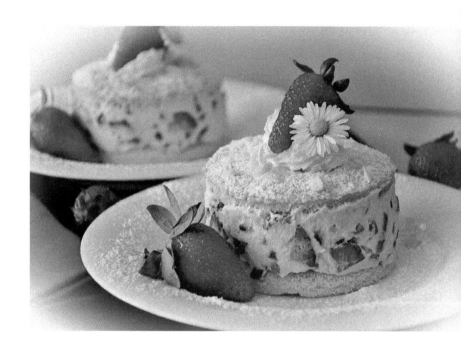

Ranch Chicken Wings

Preparation Time: 10 minutes | Cooking Time: 20 minutes | Servings: 4

Ingredients:

1 lb chicken wings

3 garlic cloves, minced

2 tbsp butter, melted

1 1/2 tbsp ranch seasoning mix

Directions:

Toss chicken wings with garlic, butter, and ranch seasoning mix.

Spray Pressure Pot multi-level air fryer basket with cooking spray.

Add chicken wings into the air fryer basket and place basket into the Pressure Pot.

Seal pot with air fryer lid and select air fry mode then set the temperature to 360° F and timer for 20 minutes. Turn wings halfway through.

Serve and enjoy.

Nutrition:

Calories 276, Fat 14.2g, Carbohydrates 0.7g, Sugar 0g, Protein 33g, Cholesterol 116mg.

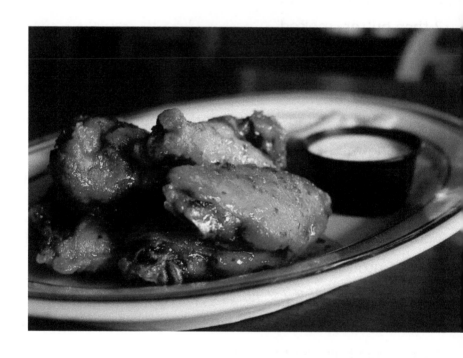

Quick-Roasted Potatoes

Preparation Time: 10 minutes | Cooking Time: 20 minutes | Servings: 4

Ingredients:

4 potatoes, cut into cubes

1 tbsp Montreal steak seasoning

1 tbsp olive oil

Directions:

Toss potatoes with seasoning and oil.

Spray Pressure Pot multi-level air fryer basket with cooking spray.

Add potatoes into the air fryer basket and place basket into the Pressure Pot.

Seal pot with air fryer lid and select air fry mode then set the temperature to 360° F and timer for 20 minutes.

Stir halfway through.

Serve and enjoy.

Nutrition:

Calories 182, Fat 3.7g, Carbohydrates 33.5g, Sugar 2.5g, Protein 3.6g, Cholesterol 0mg.

Cajun Zucchini Chips

Preparation Time: 10 minutes | Cooking Time: 16 minutes | Servings: 2

Ingredients:

1 1/4 cup zucchini slices

1 tbsp olive oil

1 tsp Cajun seasoning

Directions:

Toss zucchini slices with oil and Cajun seasoning.

Spray Pressure Pot multi-level air fryer basket with cooking spray.

Arrange zucchini slices into the air fryer basket and place basket into the Pressure Pot.

Seal pot with air fryer lid and select air fry mode then set the temperature to 370° F and timer for 16 minutes.

Turn Zucchini slices halfway through.

Serve and enjoy.

Nutrition:

Calories 179, Fat 13.9g, Carbohydrates 11.9g, Sugar 1.3g, Protein 1.3g, Cholesterol 0mg.

Macadamia Cookies

Preparation Time: 15 minutes | Cooking Time: 13 minutes | Servings: 4

Ingredients:

1 oz macadamia nuts, chopped

½ cup coconut flour

2 tablespoons butter

1 tablespoon Erythritol

1 egg, beaten

2 tablespoons flax meal

1 cup water, for cooking

Directions:

In the mixing bowl mix up macadamia nuts, coconut flour, butter, Erythritol, egg, and flax meal.

Knead the non-sticky dough.

Then cut the dough into the pieces and make balls from them.

Pour water and insert the trivet in the Pressure Pot.

Line the trivet with baking paper and put the dough balls on it.

Cook the cookies for 13 minutes on manual mode (high pressure).

When the time is over, make a quick pressure release and transfer the cookies to the plate.

Nutrition:

Calories 193, fat 15.5g, fiber 6.6g, carbs 10.1g, protein 4.8g.

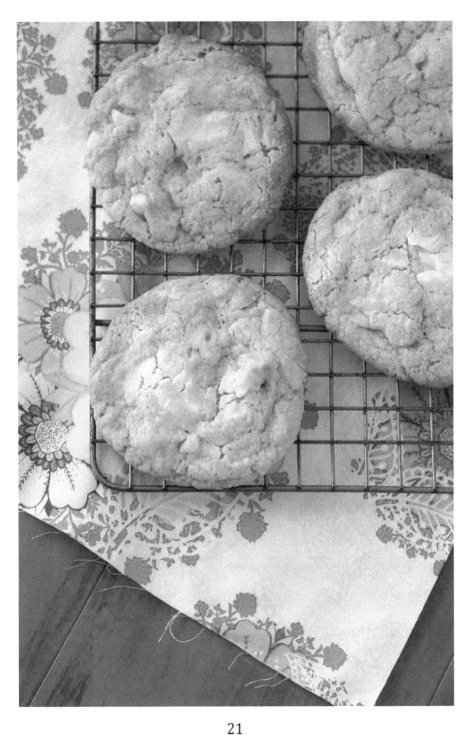

Keto Pralines

Preparation Time: 10 minutes | Cooking Time: 8 minutes | Servings: 6

Ingredients:

½ cup butter

5 tablespoons heavy cream

2 tablespoons Erythritol

¼ teaspoon xanthan gum

4 pecans, chopped

Directions:

Place the butter in the Pressure Pot and melt it on sauté mode.

Add heavy cream and Erythritol.

Stir the mixture well and sauté for 2 minutes.

After this, add xanthan gum and pecan.

Stir well and cook the mixture for 3 minutes more.

Line the baking tray with baking paper.

With the help of the spoon, place the pecan mixture in the tray in the shape of circles.

Refrigerate the pralines until they are solid.

Nutrition:

Calories 254, fat 26.6g, fiber 3.5g, carbs 4.2g, protein 1.4g.

Blueberry Crisp

Preparation Time: 10 minutes | Cooking Time: 6 minutes | Servings: 4

Ingredients:

¼ cup almonds, blended

1 teaspoon butter

1 teaspoon flax meal

1 tablespoon Erythritol

½ cup cream cheese

½ cup blueberries

1 oz peanuts, chopped

Directions:

Toss butter in the Pressure Pot and melt it on sauté mode.

Add almonds and flax meal.

Cook the mixture on sauté mode for 4 minutes. Stir it constantly.

After this, cool the mixture well.

Whisk the cream cheese with Erythritol.

Then put ½ of cream cheese mixture in the serving glasses.

Add ½ part of the almond mixture and ½ part of blueberries.

Repeat the same steps with the remaining mixtures.

Top the dessert with chopped peanuts.

Nutrition:

Calories 197, fat 17.8g, fiber 2g, carbs 6g, protein 5.6g.

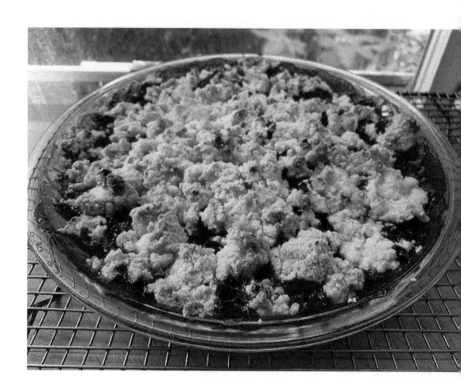

Chocolate and Bacon Bars

Preparation Time: 10 minutes | Cooking Time: 8 minutes | Servings: 6

Ingredients:

2 oz dark chocolate, chopped

4 tablespoons heavy cream

1 bacon slice, chopped

Directions:

Place the bacon in the Pressure Pot and cook it on sauté mode for 5 minutes or until it is crunchy.

Then add heavy cream and dark chocolate.

Stir the mixture well and cook for 2 minutes or until the chocolate is liquid.

Then pour the mixture into the silicone bard mold and refrigerate until solid.

Crack the dessert into the bars.

Nutrition:

calories 102, fat 7.8g, fiber 0.3g, carbs 5.9g, protein 2.1g.

Poppy Seeds Muffins

Preparation Time: 10 minutes | Cooking Time: 1: minutes | Servings: 4

Ingredients:

2 eggs, beaten

2 tablespoons butter, melted

¼ cup Erythritol

1 teaspoon vanilla extract

1 teaspoon poppy seeds

1/3 cup coconut flour

1 cup water, for cooking

Directions:

Mix up together eggs, butter, Erythritol, vanilla extract poppy seeds, and coconut flour.

Pour the batter into the muffin molds.

Pour water and insert the trivet in the Pressure Pot.

Place the muffin molds with batter on the trivet and close the lid.

Cook the muffins on manual mode (high pressure for 1: minutes.

When the time is over, make a quick pressure release and transfer the muffins to the plate.

Cool the dessert to room temperature.

Nutrition:

Calories 129, fat 9.6g, fiber 3.4g, carbs 5.8g, protein 4.3g.

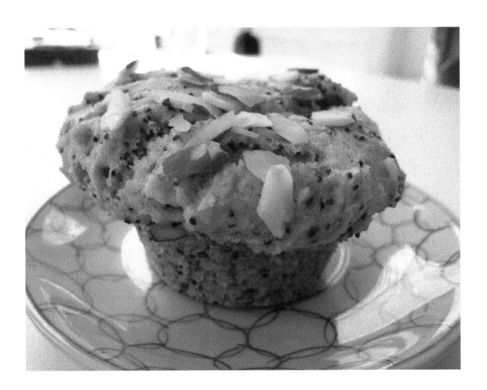

Lemon Muffins

Preparation Time: 15 minutes | Cooking Time: 10 minutes | Servings: 2

Ingredients:

1 tablespoon lemon juice

1 teaspoon lemon zest, grated

¼ teaspoon baking powder

½ cup almond meal

¼ cup heavy cream

2 teaspoons Splenda

1 cup water, for cooking

Directions:

Mix up together lemon juice, lemon zest, baking powder, almond meal, heavy cream, and Splenda.

Fill the muffin molds with lemon mixture.

Pour water and insert the steamer rack in the Pressure Pot.

Put the muffins on the steamer rack and close the lid.

Cook the muffins on manual mode (high pressure for 10 minutes.

Then allow the natural pressure release for 5 minutes.

Cool the cooked muffins well.

Nutrition:

Calories 212, fat 17.5g, fiber 3.1g, carbs 10.2g, protein 5.4g.

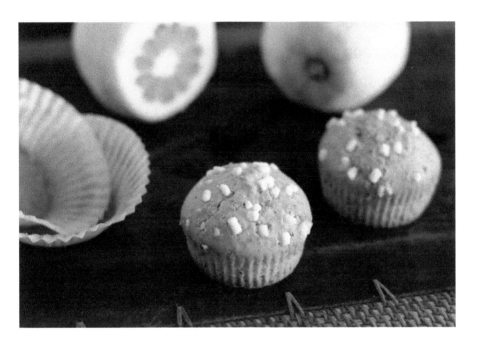

Lime Chia Seeds Pudding

Preparation Time: 5 minutes | Cooking Time: 30 minutes | Servings: 2

Ingredients:

½ cup coconut cream

1 oz chia seeds

1 tablespoon Erythritol

½ teaspoon vanilla extract

1 teaspoon lime zest, grated

Directions:

Put all ingredients in the Pressure Pot bowl and stir with the help of the spoon.

Close the lid and cook the pudding on manual mode (Low pressure for 30 minutes.

Then transfer the cooked pudding into the serving glasses.

Nutrition:

Calories 210, fat 18.7g, fiber 6.3g, carbs 9.6g, protein 3.7g.

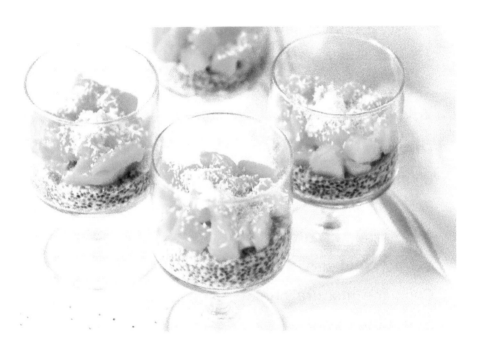

PhirniKheer with Almonds

Preparation Time: 10 minutes | Cooking Time: 6! minutes | Servings: 3

Ingredients:

½ cup whipped cream

½ teaspoon ground cardamom

½ cup of organic almond milk

1 scoop stevia

¼ cup coconut flour

¼ teaspoon vanilla extract

Directions:

Pour whipped cream and almond milk into the Pressure Pot.

Add ground cardamom, coconut flour, and vanilla extract. Add stevia and stir the liquid well.

Cook the mixture on sauté mode for 5 minutes. Stir it from time to time.

Then switch the Pressure Pot on manual mode (low pressure).

Cook the meal for 1 hour.

Stir the cooked kheer well and pour into the serving glasses.

Nutrition:

Calories 114, fat 8.5g, fiber 3.8g, carbs 6.9g, protein 2.1g.

Blueberry Cream

Preparation time: 24 minutes | Cooking Time: 40 minutes | Servings: 6

Ingredients:

2 cups blueberries

2 tbsp. Swerve

2 tbsp. Water

1 tsp. Vanilla extract

Juice of ½ lemon

Directions:

Take a bowl and mix all the ingredients and whisk well.

Divide this into 6 ramekins, put them in the air fryer, and cook at 340°f for 20 minutes.

Cooldown and serve

Nutrition:

Calories 123, Fat 2g, Fiber 2g, Carbs 4g, Protein 3g.

Coconut Donuts

Preparation time: 20 minutes | Cooking Time: 40 minutes | Servings: 4

Ingredients:

8 oz. Coconut flour

4 oz. Coconut milk

1 egg, whisked

2 tbsp. Stevia

2 ½ tbsp. Butter; melted

1 tsp. Baking powder

Directions:

Take a bowl and mix all the ingredients and whisk well.

Shape donuts from this mix and place them in your air fryer's basket and cook at 370°f for 15 minutes.

Serve warm

Nutrition:

Calories 190, Fat 12g, Fiber 1g, Carbs 4g, Protein 6g.

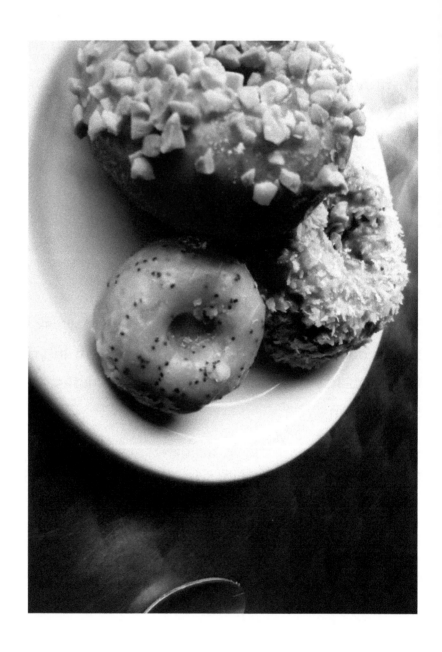

Turkey Bowls

Preparation time: 10 minutes | Cooking Time: 20 minutes | Servings: 2

Ingredients:

1 tablespoon olive oil

2 cups okra, sliced

½ cup chicken stock

2 cups yellow bell pepper, chopped

A pinch of salt and black pepper

1 turkey breast, skinless, boneless, and cubed

2 tablespoons oregano, chopped

1 tablespoon thyme, chopped

½ cup balsamic vinegar

Directions:

Set the Pressure Pot on sauté mode, add the oil, heat it, add the turkey and brown for 5 minutes.

Add the okra and the rest of the Ingredients put the lid on and cook on High for 15 minutes.

Release the pressure naturally for 10 minutes, divide the mix into bowls and serve for breakfast.

Nutrition:

Calories 171, fat 8.2g, fiber 2.6g, carbs 7.8g, protein 3.9g.

Cheesy Tomato and Radish Salad

Preparation time: 10 minutes | Cooking Time: 10 minutes | Servings: 4

Ingredients:

¼ cup radishes, sliced

1 pound cherry tomatoes, halved

1 tablespoon basil, chopped

1 tablespoon olive oil

1 tablespoon chives, chopped

½ cup mozzarella, shredded

A pinch of salt and black pepper

Directions:

In your Pressure Pot, mix the radishes with the tomatoes and the rest of the ingredients except the mozzarella, and toss.

Sprinkle the cheese on top, put the lid on, and cook on High for 10 minutes.

Release the pressure naturally for 10 minutes, divide the salad into bowls and serve for breakfast.

Nutrition:

Calories 62, fat 4.4g, fiber 1.5g, carbs 4.9g, protein 2.1g.

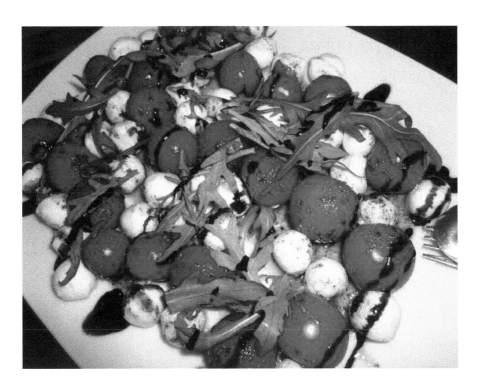

Pork and Kale Hash

Preparation time: 10 minutes | Cooking Time: 15 minutes | Servings: 4

Ingredients:

1 tablespoon avocado oil

1 spring onion, chopped

2 cups pork meat, ground

2 garlic cloves, minced

½ cup beef stock

A pinch of salt and black pepper

1 pound kale, torn

Directions:

Set your Pressure Pot on sauté mode, add the oil, heat it, add the onion, garlic, and the meat, and brown for 5 minutes.

Add the rest of the ingredients, toss, put the lid on, and cook on High for 10 minutes.

Release the pressure naturally for 10 minutes, divide the mix between plates and serve.

Nutrition:

Calories 66, fat 5.3g, fiber 2g, carbs 6.5g, protein 3.8g.

Sweet Zucchini Mix

Preparation time: 10 minutes | Cooking Time: 10 minutes | Servings: 4

Ingredients:

1 and ½ cups of coconut cream

1 teaspoon nutmeg, ground

4 zucchinis, sliced

2 tablespoons swerve

¼ cup walnuts, chopped

Directions:

In your Pressure Pot, combine the cream with the zucchinis and the rest of the ingredients, put the lid on and cook on High for 10 minutes.

Release the pressure naturally for 10 minutes, divide the mix into bowls and serve.

Nutrition:

Calories 83, fat 8.2g, fiber 2.8g, carbs 7.6g, protein 4.3g.

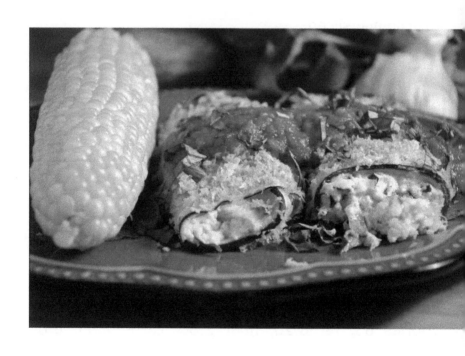

Turkey Omelet

Preparation time: 10 minutes | Cooking Time: 15 minutes | Servings: 4

Ingredients:

1 cup turkey breast, skinless, boneless and cut into strips

1 tomato, chopped

2 bacon slices, cooked and crumbled

4 eggs, whisked

1 small avocado, pitted, peeled, and chopped

A pinch of salt and black pepper

2 tablespoons olive oil

Directions:

Set your Pressure Pot on sauté mode, add half of the oil, heat it, add the meat, and cook for 5 minutes.

Add the rest of the ingredients, toss, spread the mix into the pot, put the lid on, and cook on High for 10 minutes.

Release the pressure naturally for 10 minutes, divide the omelet between plates and serve.

Nutrition:

Calories 228, fat 21.2g, fiber 3.6g, carbs 5.3g, protein 6.6g.

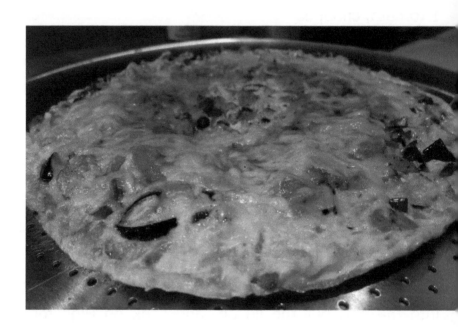

Strawberries and Nuts Salad

Preparation time: 10 minutes | Cooking Time: 10 minutes | Servings: 4

Ingredients:

½ cup almonds, chopped

½ cup walnuts, chopped

2 cups strawberries, halved

1 tablespoon stevia

½ teaspoon nutmeg, ground

1 cup coconut cream

Directions:

In your Pressure Pot, mix the strawberries with the cream and the rest of the ingredients, put the lid on and cook on Low for 10 minutes.

Release the pressure naturally for 10 minutes.

Divide the mix into bowls and serve.

Nutrition:

Calories 328, fat 29.8g, fiber 5.4g, carbs 7.6g, protein 8.1g.

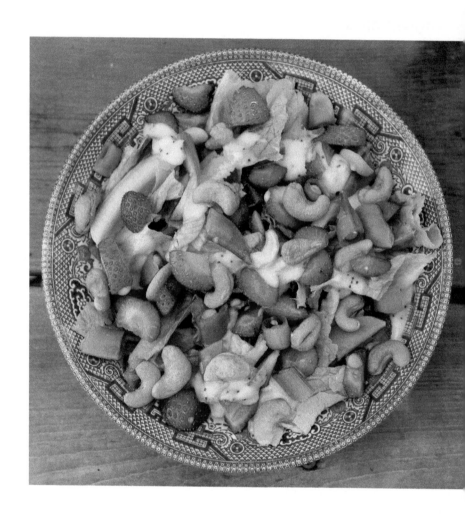

Eggs, Leeks, and Turkey Mix

Preparation time: 10 minutes | Cooking Time: 15 minutes | Servings: 4

Ingredients:

2 leeks, chopped

½ cup chicken stock

2 tablespoons olive oil

2 garlic cloves, minced

8 eggs, whisked

1 turkey breast, skinless, boneless and cut into strips

Directions:

Set your Pressure Pot on Sauté mode, add the oil, heat it, add the leeks, garlic, and the meat, and brown for 5 minutes.

Add the rest of the ingredients, toss, put the lid on, and cook on High for 10 minutes.

Release the pressure naturally for 10 minutes.

Divide the mix between plates and serve.

Nutrition:

Calories 216, fat 16g, fiber 0.8g, carbs 7.6g, protein 11.9g.

Sweet Berries Bowls

Preparation time: 10 minutes | Cooking Time: 12 minutes | Servings: 6

Ingredients:

3 tablespoons coconut flakes, unsweetened

1 cup strawberries

1 cup blackberries

2 cups almond milk

1 teaspoon vanilla extract

1 teaspoon swerve

Directions:

In your Pressure Pot, mix the berries with the coconut and the rest of the ingredients, put the lid on and cook on Low for 12 minutes.

Release the pressure naturally for 10 minutes.

Divide the mix into bowls and serve.

Nutrition:

Calories 213, fat 20.1g, fiber 3.7g, carbs 6.7g, protein 2.4g

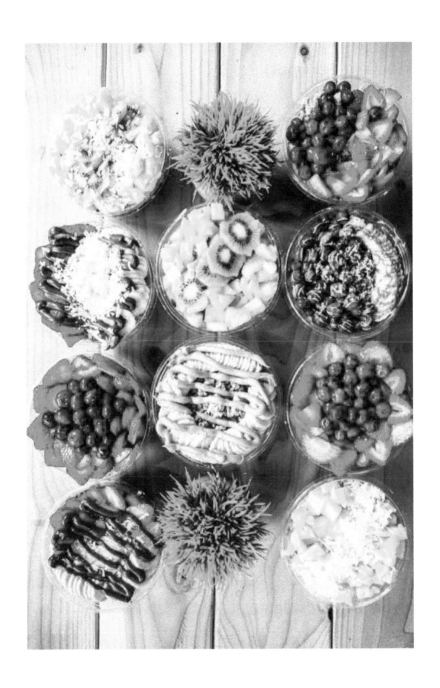

Mushroom and Okra Omelet

Preparation time: 10 minutes | Cooking Time: 1! minutes | Servings: 2

Ingredients:

1 pound white mushrooms, sliced

2 spring onions, chopped

2 garlic cloves, minced

1 tablespoon avocado oil

2 chili peppers, minced

1 cup okra

½ cup cilantro, chopped

4 eggs, whisked

Directions:

Set your Pressure Pot on sauté mode, add the oil, heat it, add the onions and garlic and sauté for 2 minutes.

Add the mushrooms and sauté for 2 minutes more.

Add the rest of the ingredients, toss, spread the mix into the Pressure Pot, put the lid on, and cook on High for 10 minutes.

Release the pressure naturally for 10 minutes, divide the omelet between plates and serve.

Nutrition:

Calories 108, fat 5.2g, fiber 2.4g, carbs 4.7g, protein 9.9g.

Easy Salmon Bites

Preparation Time: 10 minutes | Cooking Time: 12 minutes | Servings: 4

Ingredients:

1 lb salmon fillets, boneless and cut into chunks

2 tsp olive oil

1/4 tsp cayenne

1/2 tsp chili powder

1 tsp dried dill

Pepper

Salt

Directions:

Add salmon and remaining ingredients into the large bowl and toss well.

Spray Pressure Pot multi-level air fryer basket with cooking spray.

Add salmon chunks into the air fryer basket and place basket into the Pressure Pot.

Seal pot with air fryer lid and select air fry mode then set the temperature to 350° F and timer for 12 minutes.

Turn salmon chunks halfway through.

Serve and enjoy.

Nutrition:

Calories 172, Fat 9.4g, Carbohydrates 0.4g, Sugar 0g, Protein 22.1g, Cholesterol 50mg.

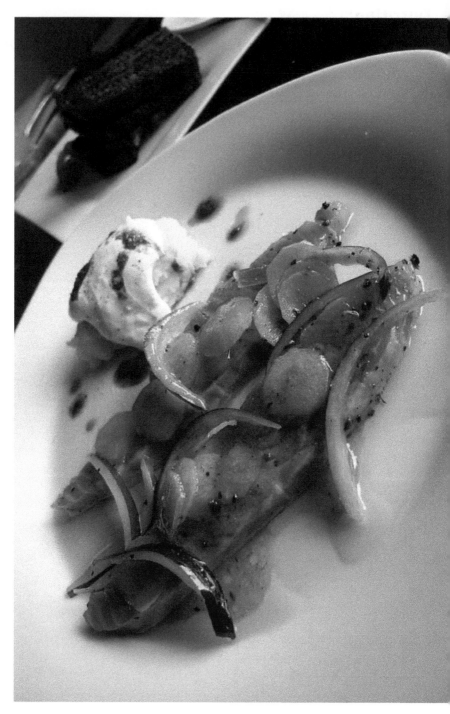

Air Fried Cauliflower Bites

Preparation Time: 10 minutes | Cooking Time: 14 minutes | Servings: 4

Ingredients:

1 lb cauliflower florets

1 1/2 tsp garlic powder

1 tbsp olive oil

1 tsp ground coriander

1 tsp dried rosemary

Pepper

Salt

Directions:

Add cauliflower florets into the large bowl. Add remaining ingredients and toss well.

Spray Pressure Pot multi-level air fryer basket with cooking spray.

Add cauliflower florets into the air fryer basket and place basket into the Pressure Pot.

Seal pot with air fryer lid and select air fry mode then set the temperature to 400° F and timer for 14 minutes. Stir halfway through.

Serve and enjoy.

Nutrition:

Calories 63, Fat 3.7g, Carbohydrates 7g, Sugar 3g Protein 2.4g, Cholesterol 0mg.

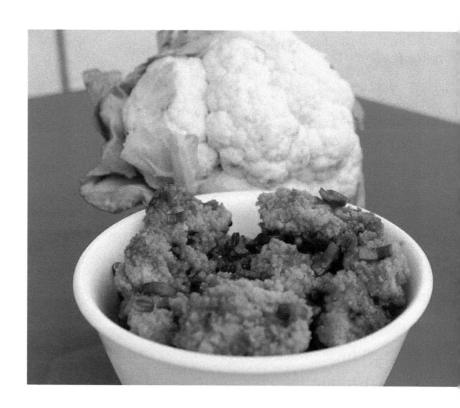

Air Fried Simple Tofu Bites

Preparation Time: 10 minutes | Cooking Time: 20 minutes | Servings: 4

Ingredients:

10 oz tofu, cut into cubes

1 1/2 tbsp dried rosemary

1 tsp vinegar

2 tsp olive oil

Pepper

Salt

Directions:

Add tofu and remaining ingredients into the large bowl and toss well.

Spray Pressure Pot multi-level air fryer basket with cooking spray.

Add tofu cubes into the air fryer basket and place basket into the Pressure Pot.

Seal pot with air fryer lid and select air fry mode then set the temperature to 350° F and timer for 20 minutes. Stir halfway through.

Serve and enjoy.

Nutrition:

Calories 74, Fat 5.5g, Carbohydrates 2g, Sugar 0.4g, Protein 5.9g, Cholesterol 0mg.

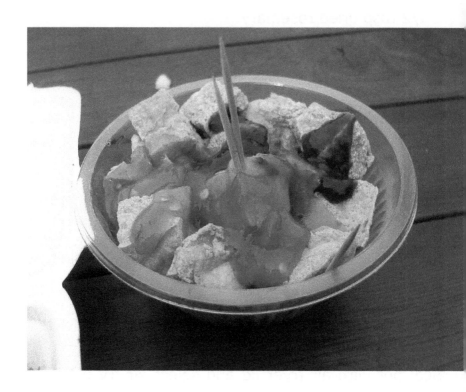

Roasted Almonds

Preparation Time: 10 minutes | Cooking Time: 5 minutes | Servings: 4

Ingredients:

1 cup almonds

1/4 tsp cayenne

1 tsp olive oil

Pepper

Salt

Directions:

In a bowl, toss almonds with cayenne, oil, pepper, and salt.

Spray Pressure Pot multi-level air fryer basket with cooking spray.

Add almonds into the air fryer basket and place basket into the Pressure Pot.

Seal pot with air fryer lid and select air fry mode then set the temperature to 350° F and timer for 5 minutes. Stir after 3 minutes.

Serve and enjoy.

Nutrition:

Calories 148, Fat 13.1g, Carbohydrates 5.2g, Sugar 1g, Protein 5g, Cholesterol 0mg.

Healthy Eggplant Chips

Preparation Time: 10 minutes | Cooking Time: 30 minutes | Servings: 2

Ingredients:

1 eggplant, sliced 1/4-inch thick

2 tbsp rosemary, chopped

1/2 cup parmesan cheese, grated

Pepper

Salt

Directions:

Add eggplant slices, cheese, rosemary, pepper, and salt into the mixing bowl and toss well.

Place the dehydrating tray in a multi-level air fryer basket and place basket in the Pressure Pot.

Arrange eggplant slices on the dehydrating tray.

Seal pot with air fryer lid and select air fry mode then set the temperature to 400° F and timer for 30 minutes.

Turn eggplant slices halfway through.

Serve and enjoy.

Nutrition:

Calories 141, Fat 5.7g, Carbohydrates 16.4g, Sugar 6.9g, Protein 9.6g, Cholesterol 16mg.

Crispy Roasted Cashews

Preparation Time: 10 minutes | Cooking Time: 6 minutes | Servings: 3

Ingredients:

1 cup cashews

1/4 tsp onion powder

1/4 tsp garlic powder

1/2 tsp nutritional yeast

1 tbsp rice flour

1 tbsp olive oil

Pepper

Salt

Directions:

Add cashews and remaining ingredients into the large bowl and toss well.

Place the dehydrating tray in a multi-level air fryer basket and place basket in the Pressure Pot.

Spread cashews on a dehydrating tray.

Seal pot with air fryer lid and select air fry mode then set the temperature to 350° F and timer for 6 minutes. Stir halfway through.

Serve and enjoy.

Nutrition:

Calories 318, Fat 25.9g, Carbohydrates 18.2g, Sugar 2.4g, Protein 7.5g, Cholesterol 0mg.

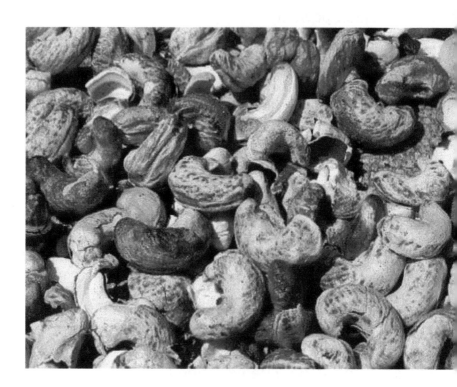

Fried Bananas with Chocolate Sauce

Preparation time: 10 minutes | Cooking Time: 10 minutes | Servings: 2

Ingredients:

1 large egg

¼ cup cornstarch

¼ cup plain bread crumbs

3 bananas, halved crosswise

Cooking oil

Chocolate sauce (see ingredient tip

Directions:

Preparing the ingredients. In a small bowl, beat the egg.

In another bowl, place the cornstarch. Place the bread crumbs in a third bowl.

Dip the bananas in the cornstarch, then the egg, and then the bread crumbs.

Spray the instant crisp air fryer basket with cooking oil.

Place the bananas in the basket and spray them with cooking oil.

Air frying. Close the air fryer lid. Cook for 5 minutes.

Open the instant crisp air fryer and flip the bananas.

Cook for an additional 2 minutes. Transfer the bananas to plates.

Drizzle the chocolate sauce over the bananas, and serve.

You can make your chocolate sauce using 2 tablespoons of milk and ¼ cup chocolate chips.

Heat a saucepan over medium-high heat. Add the milk and stir for 1 to 2 minutes.

Add the chocolate chips.

Stir for 2 minutes, or until the chocolate has melted.

Nutrition:

Calories 203, Fat 6g, Protein 3g, Fiber 3g.

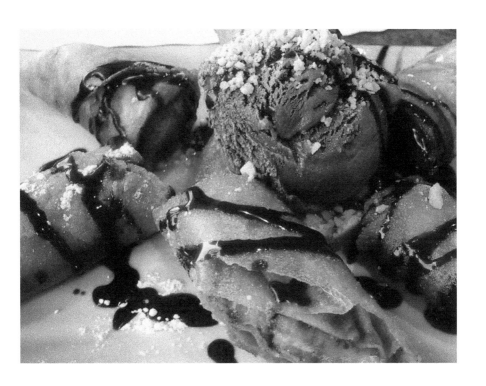

Apple Hand Pies

Preparation time: 5 minutes | Cooking Time: 8 minutes | Servings: 6

Ingredients:

15-ounces no-sugar-added apple pie filling

1 store-bought crust

Directions:

Preparing the Ingredients.

Layout pie crust and slice into equal-sized squares.

Place 2 tbsp. Filling into each square and seal crust with a fork.

Air frying. Place into the instant crisp air fryer.

Close the air fryer lid.

Select bake set the temperature to 390°f and set the time to 8 minutes until golden in color.

Select start to begin.

Nutrition:

Calories 278, Fat 10g, Protein 5g, Sugar 4g.

Blueberry Lemon Muffins

Preparation time: 5 minutes | Cooking Time: 10 minutes | Servings: 12

Ingredients:

1 tsp. Vanilla

Juice and zest of 1 lemon

2 eggs

1 c. Blueberries

½ c. Cream

¼ c. Avocado oil

½ c. Monk fruit

2 ½ c. Almond flour

Directions:

Preparing the ingredients. Mix monk fruit and flour.

In another bowl, mix vanilla, egg, lemon juice, and cream.

Add mixtures together and blend well.

Spoon batter into cupcake holders.

Air frying. Place in the instant crisp air fryer.

Close the air fryer lid. Select bake set the temperature to 320°f and set the time to 10 minutes.

Select start to begin checking at 6 minutes to ensure you don't overbake them.

Nutrition:

Calories 317, Fat 11g, Protein 3g, Sugar 5g.

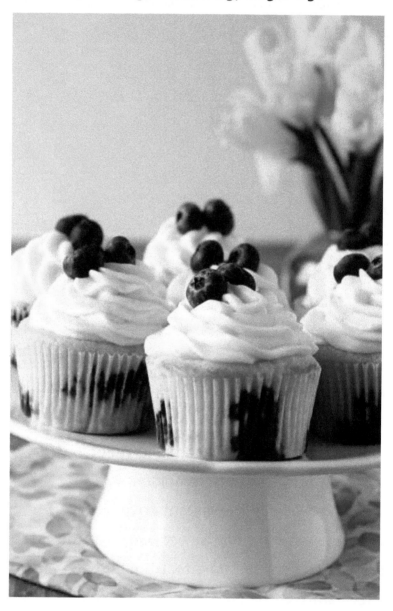

Sweet Cream Cheese Wontons

Preparation time: 5 minutes | Cooking Time: 5 minutes | Servings: 16

Ingredients:

1 egg mixed with a bit of water

Wonton wrappers

½ c. Powdered erythritol

8 ounces softened cream cheese

Olive oil

Directions:

Preparing the ingredients.

Mix sweetener and cream cheese together.

Layout 4 wontons at a time and cover with a dish towel to prevent drying out.

Place ½ of a teaspoon of cream cheese mixture into each wrapper.

Dip finger into egg/water mixture and fold diagonally to form a triangle. Seal edges well.

Repeat with remaining ingredients.

Air frying. Place filled wontons into the instant crisp air fryer.

Close the air fryer lid. Select bake and cook 5 minutes at 400° F, shaking halfway through cooking.

Nutrition:

Calories 303, Fat 3g, Protein 0.5g, Sugar 4g.

Air Fryer Cinnamon Rolls

Preparation time: 15 minutes | Cooking Time: 5 minutes | Servings: 8

Ingredients:

1 ½ tbsp. Cinnamon

¾ c. Brown sugar

¼ c. Melted coconut oil

1-pound frozen bread dough, thawed

Glaze:

½ tsp. Vanilla

1 ¼ c. Powdered erythritol

2 tbsp. Softened ghee

Ounces softened cream cheese

Directions:

Preparing the ingredients. Layout bread dough and roll it out into a rectangle.

Brush melted ghee over the dough and leave a 1-inch border along the edges.

Mix cinnamon and sweetener and then sprinkle over dough.

Roll dough tightly and slice into 8 pieces. Let sit 1-2 hours to rise.

To make the glaze, simply mix ingredients together till smooth.

Air frying. Once rolls rise, place into an instant crisp air fryer.

Close the air fryer lid. Select bake and cook for 5 minutes at 350° F.

Serve rolls drizzled in cream cheese glaze.

Enjoy!

Nutrition:

Calories 390, Fat 8g, Protein 1g, Sugar 7g.

Bread Pudding with Cranberry

Preparation time: 5 minutes | Cooking Time: 45 minutes | Servings: 4

Ingredients:

1-1/2 cups milk

2-1/2 eggs

1/2 cup cranberries1 teaspoon butter

1/4 cup and 2 tablespoons white sugar

1/4 cup golden raisins

1/8 teaspoon ground cinnamon

3/4 cup heavy whipping cream

3/4 teaspoon lemon zest

3/4 teaspoon kosher salt

3/4 French baguettes, cut into 2-inch slices

3/8 vanilla bean, split and seeds scraped away

Directions:

Preparing the ingredients.

Lightly grease the baking pan of the instant crisp air fryer with cooking spray.

Spread baguette slices, cranberries, and raisins.

In a blender, blend well vanilla bean, cinnamon, salt, lemon zest, eggs, sugar, and cream.

Pour over baguette slices. Let it soak for an hour.

Cover pan with foil.

Air frying. Close the air fryer lid.

Select bake and cook for 35 minutes, cook at 330°f.

Let it rest for 10 minutes.

Serve and enjoy.

Nutrition:

Calories 581, Fat 23.8g, Protein 15.8g, Sugar 7g.

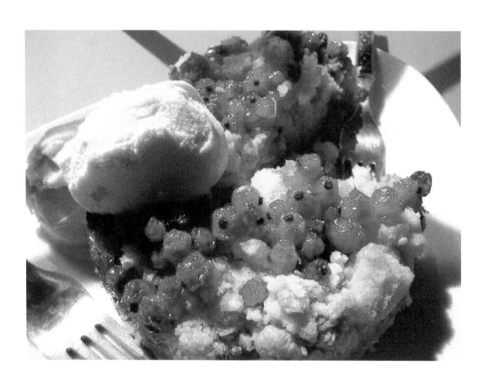

Black and White Brownies

Preparation time: 10 minutes | Cooking Time: 20 minutes | Servings: 8

Ingredients:

1 egg

¼ cup brown sugar

2 tablespoons white sugar

2 tablespoons safflower oil

1 teaspoon vanilla

¼ cup of cocoa powder

⅓ cup all-purpose flour

¼ cup white chocolate chips

Nonstick baking spray with flour

Directions:

Preparing the ingredients. In a medium bowl, beat the egg with brown sugar and white sugar.

Beat in the oil and vanilla.

Add the cocoa powder and flour and stir just until combined.

Fold in the white chocolate chips.

Spray a 6-by-6-by-2-inch baking pan with nonstick spray.

Spoon the brownie batter into the pan.

Air frying. Close the air fryer lid.

Select bake, and bake for 20 minutes or until the brownies are set when lightly touched with a finger.

Let cool for 30 minutes before slicing to serve.

Nutrition:

Calories 81, Fat 4g, Protein 1g, Fiber 1g.

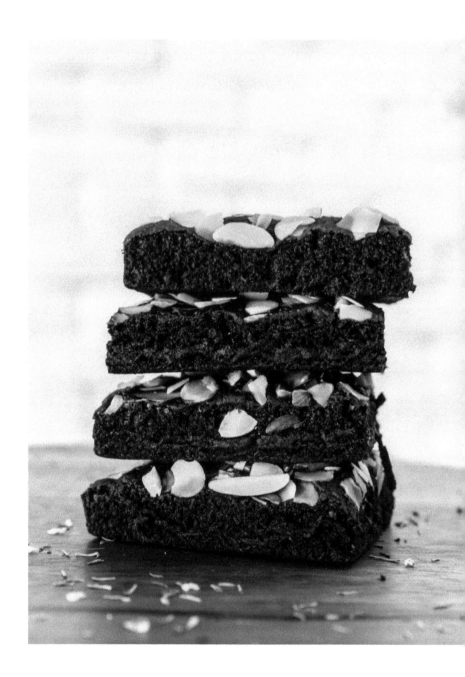

Oats Cookies

Preparation Time: 10 minutes | Cooking Time: 15 minutes | Servings: 3

Ingredients:

1 cup quick oats

2 tbsp milk

2 ripe bananas, mashed

2 tbsp coconut shredded

Directions:

Add all ingredients into the mixing bowl and mix until combined.

Line Pressure Pot air fryer basket with parchment paper or foil.

Spoon cookie dough onto parchment paper.

Place air fryer basket in the pot.

Seal air fryer basket with air fryer lid and select bake mode and cook at 350° F for 15 minutes.

Serve and enjoy.

Nutrition:

Calories 198, Fat 3.6g, Carbohydrates 38.8g, Sugar 12g, Protein 4.9g, Cholesterol 1mg.

Baked Pineapple Slices

Preparation Time: 10 minutes | Cooking Time: 1(
minutes | Servings: 2

Ingredients:

2 pineapple slices

1/2 tsp cinnamon

1/4 cup brown sugar

Directions:

Add cinnamon and brown sugar in a zip-lock bag an(
mix well.

Add pineapple slices in the zip-lock bag and shake wel
to coat.

Seal bag and place in the fridge for 30 minutes.

Spray Pressure Pot air fryer basket with cooking spray.

Place pineapple slices in the air fryer basket and plac(
basket in the pot.

Seal the pot with an air fryer lid and select bake mod(
and cook at 350° F for 20 minutes.

Turn pineapple slices halfway through.

Serve and enjoy.

Nutrition:

Calories 152, Fat 0.2g, Carbohydrates 39.9g, Suga
33.9g, Protein 0.9g, Cholesterol 0mg.

Cocoa and Nuts Bombs

Preparation time: 13 minutes | Cooking Time: 40 minutes | Servings: 12

Ingredients:

2 cups macadamia nuts; chopped.

¼ cup of cocoa powder

1/3 cup swerve

4 tbsp. Coconut oil; melted

1 tsp. Vanilla extract

Directions:

Take a bowl and mix all the ingredients and whisk well.

Shape medium balls out of this mix, place them in your air fryer, and cook at 300°f for 8 minutes.

Serve cold

Nutrition:

Calories 120, Fat 12g, Fiber 1g, Carbs 2g, Protein 1g.

Cream Cheese and Zucchinis Bars

Preparation time: 25 minutes | Cooking Time: 40 minutes | Servings: 12

Ingredients:

3 oz. Zucchini, shredded

4 oz. Cream cheese

6 eggs

2 tbsp. Erythritol

3 tbsp. Coconut oil; melted

2 tsp. Vanilla extract

½ tsp. Baking powder

Directions:

In a bowl, combine all the ingredients and whisk well.

Pour this into a baking dish that fits your air fryer lined with parchment paper, introduce in the fryer and cook at 320°f, bake for 15 minutes.

Slice and serve cold

Nutrition:

Calories 178, Fat 8g, Fiber 3g, Carbs 4g, Protein 5g.

Chocolate Strawberry Cups

Preparation time: 15 minutes | Cooking Time: 40 minutes | Servings: 8

Ingredients:

16 strawberries; halved

2 cups chocolate chips; melted

2 tbsp. Coconut oil

Directions:

In a pan that fits your air fryer, mix the strawberries with the oil and the melted chocolate chips, toss gently, put the pan in the air fryer, and cook at 340°f for 10 minutes.

Divide into cups and serve cold

Nutrition:

Calories 162, Fat 5g, Fiber 3g, Carbs 5g, Protein 6g.

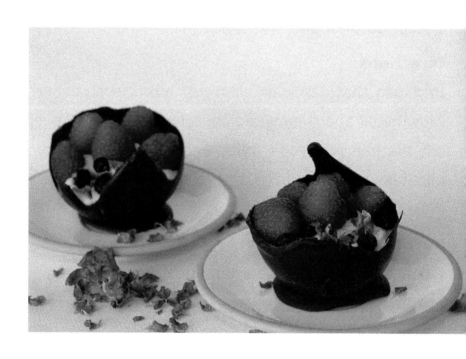

Sponge Ricotta Cake

Preparation time: 35 minutes | Cooking Time: 40 minutes | Servings: 8

Ingredients:

3 eggs, whisked

1 cup almond flour

1 cup ricotta, soft

1/3 swerve

7 tbsp. Ghee; melted

1 tsp. Baking powder

Cooking spray

Directions:

In a bowl, combine all the ingredients except the cooking spray and stir them very well.

Grease a cake pan that fits the air fryer with the cooking spray and pours the cake mix inside.

Put the pan in the fryer and cook at 350°f for 30 minutes

Cool the cake down, slice, and serve.

Nutrition:

Calories 210, Fat 12g, Fiber 3g, Carbs 6g, Protein 9g.

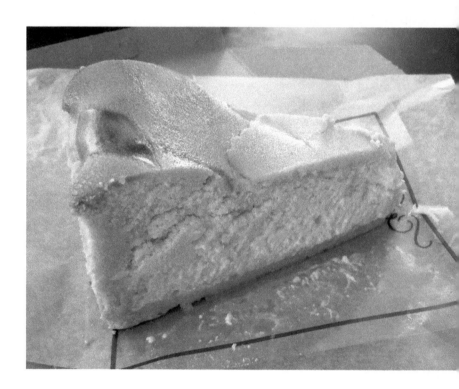

Mini Lava Cakes

Preparation time: 30 minutes | Cooking Time: 40 minutes | Servings: 4

Ingredients:

3 oz. Dark chocolate; melted

2 eggs, whisked

¼ cup coconut oil; melted

1 tbsp. Almond flour

2 tbsp. Swerve

¼ tsp. Vanilla extract

Cooking spray

Directions:

In a bowl, combine all the ingredients except the cooking spray and whisk well.

Divide this into 4 ramekins greased with cooking spray, put them in the fryer, and cook at 360°f for 20 minutes

Nutrition:

Calories 161, Fat 12g, Fiber 1g, Carbs 4g, Protein 7g.

Lemon Cookies

Preparation time: 30 minutes | Cooking Time: 40 minutes | Servings: 12

Ingredients:

¼ cup cashew butter, soft

1 egg, whisked

¾ cup swerve

1 cup coconut cream

Juice of 1 lemon

1 tsp. Baking powder

1 tsp. Lemon peel, grated

Directions:

In a bowl, combine all the ingredients gradually and stir well.

Spoon balls this on a cookie sheet lined with parchment paper and flatten them.

Put the cookie sheet in the fryer and cook at 350°f for 20 minutes.

Serve the cookies cold

Nutrition:

Calories 121, Fat 5g, Fiber 1g, Carbs 4g, Protein 2g.

Blackberry and Chocolate Cream

Preparation time: 20 minutes | Cooking Time: 40 minutes | Servings: 6

Ingredients:

1 cup blackberries

2 eggs

¼ cup chocolate; melted

½ cup heavy cream

½ cup ghee; melted

1 tbsp. Stevia

2 tsp. Baking powder

Directions:

Take a bowl and mix the blackberries with the rest of the ingredients, whisk well.

Divide into ramekins, put them in the fryer, and cook at 340°f for 15 minutes.

Serve cold!

Nutrition:

Calories 150, Fat 2g, Fiber 2g, Carbs 4g, Protein 7g.

Cocoa Cake

Preparation time: 25 minutes | Cooking Time: 40 minutes | Servings: 8

Ingredients:

2 egg

¼ cup coconut milk

4 tbsp. Almond flour

1 tbsp. Cocoa powder

3 tbsp. Swerve

3 tbsp. Coconut oil; melted

½ tsp. Baking powder

Directions:

Take a bowl and mix all the ingredients and stir well.

Pour this into a cake pan that fits the air fryer, put the pan in the machine, and cook at 340°f for 20 minutes.

Nutrition:

Calories 191, Fat 12g, Fiber 2g, Carbs 4g, Protein 6g.

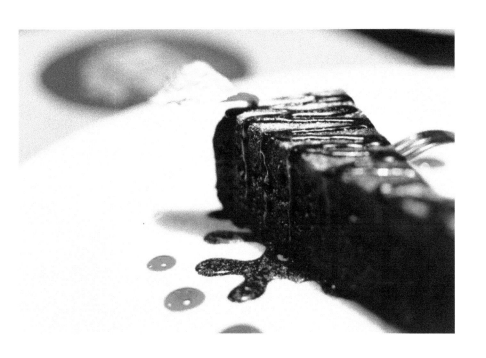

Currant Pudding

Preparation time: 25 minutes | Cooking Time: 4(minutes | Servings: 6

Ingredients:

1 cup red currants, blended

1 cup coconut cream

1 cup black currants, blended

3 tbsp. Stevia

Directions:

In a bowl, combine all the ingredients and stir well.

Divide into ramekins, put them in the fryer and cook at 340°F for 20 minutes

Serve the pudding cold.

Nutrition:

Calories 200, Fat 4g, Fiber 2g, Carbs 4g, Protein 6g.

Fudgy Brownie Pots

Preparation Time: 10 minutes | Cooking Time: 25 minutes | Servings: 2

Ingredients:

1 egg

1/4 tsp baking powder

1/3 cup cocoa powder

1/3 cup all-purpose flour

1/4 tsp vanilla

1/2 cup sugar

4 tbsp butter, melted

1/8 tsp salt

Directions:

In a small bowl, whisk together melted butter and sugar until well combined.

Add egg and vanilla and stir until combined.

In a medium bowl, mix flour, cocoa powder, baking powder, and salt.

Add egg mixture into the flour mixture and mix until combined.

Pour batter into the two ramekins.

Place the dehydrating tray in a multi-level air fryer basket and place basket in the Pressure Pot.

Place ramekins on a dehydrating tray.

Seal pot with air fryer lid and select bake mode then set the temperature to 350° F and timer for 25 minutes.

Serve and enjoy.

Nutrition:

Calories 532, Fat 27.3g, Carbohydrates 74.3g, Sugar 50.6g, Protein 7.8g, Cholesterol 143mg.

Peanut Butter Cookies

Preparation Time: 10 minutes | Cooking Time: 10 minutes | Servings: 12

Ingredients:

1 egg

1 cup peanut butter

1/2 cup erythritol

Directions:

In a mixing bowl, mix egg, peanut butter, and sweetener until a soft mixture is formed.

Place the dehydrating tray in a multi-level air fryer basket and place basket in the Pressure Pot.

Line dehydrating tray with parchment paper.

Make cookies from the mixture and place some cookies on the dehydrating tray.

Seal pot with air fryer lid and select bake mode then set the temperature to 350 F and timer for 12 minutes.

Bake remaining cookies using the same method.

Serve and enjoy.

Nutrition:

Calories 132, Fat 11.2g, Carbohydrates 14.3g, Sugar 12.1g, Protein 5.8g, Cholesterol 14mg.

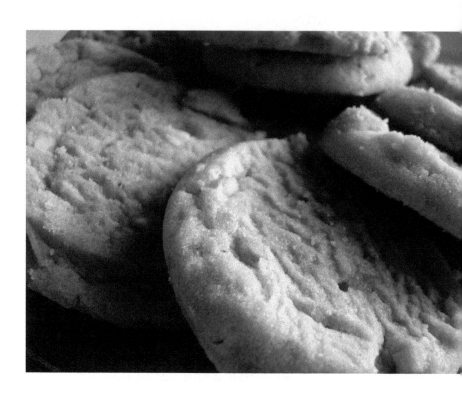

Chewy Brownies

Preparation Time: 10 minutes | Cooking Time: 30 minutes | Servings: 6

Ingredients:

2 eggs

1/2 cup walnuts, chopped

1/4 cup all-purpose flour

1 cup brown sugar

2 tsp vanilla

1/4 cup cocoa powder

1/2 cup butter, melted

1/8 tsp salt

Directions:

Spray a baking dish with cooking spray and set it aside.

In a bowl, whisk eggs with vanilla, butter, and cocoa powder.

Add flour, walnuts, sugar, and salt and stir until well combined.

Pour batter into the prepared baking dish.

Place steam rack into the Pressure Pot then places baking dish on top of the rack.

Seal pot with air fryer lid and select air fry mode then set the temperature to 320° F and timer for 30 minutes.

Serve and enjoy.

Nutrition:

Calories 344, Fat 23.5g, Carbohydrates 31g, Sugar 23.9g, Protein 5.7g, Cholesterol 95mg.

Lemon Pound Cake

Preparation Time: 10 minutes | Cooking Time: 30 minutes | Servings: 6

Ingredients:

4 eggs

2/3 cup yogurt

1 tsp vanilla

2 tbsp fresh lemon juice

1 tbsp lemon zest, grated

1 cup Swerve

1/2 cup butter, softened

1 tsp baking powder

1 1/2 cups all-purpose flour

1/2 tsp salt

Directions:

Spray Bundt cake pan with cooking spray and set aside.

In a medium bowl, mix flour, baking powder, and salt.

In a mixing bowl, beat together butter and sweetener until creamy.

Add eggs and beat until well combined.

Add flour mixture, vanilla, yogurt, lemon juice, and lemon zest and blend until smooth.

Pour batter into the prepared cake pan.

Place steam rack into the Pressure Pot then places the cake pan on top of the rack.

Seal pot with air fryer lid and select air fry mode then set the temperature to 320° F and timer for 30 minutes. Serve and enjoy.

Nutrition:

Calories 316, Fat 19g, Carbohydrates 27.1g, Sugar 2.5g, Protein 8.7g, Cholesterol 151mg.

Sugar Cookies

Preparation Time: 10 minutes | Cooking Time: 12 minutes | Servings: 6

Ingredients:

1 egg yolk

1/4 tsp baking soda

1/2 cup + 2 tbsp all-purpose flour

1/2 tsp vanilla

1/3 cup granulated sugar

1/4 cup butter, melted

Pinch of salt

Directions:

In a bowl, stir together the egg yolk, vanilla, sugar, and butter until well combined.

Add flour, baking soda, and flour and mix until dough is formed.

Place the dehydrating tray in a multi-level air fryer basket and place basket in the Pressure Pot.

Line dehydrating tray with parchment paper.

Make cookies from mixture and place on dehydrating tray.

Seal pot with air fryer lid and select bake mode then set the temperature to 350° F and timer for 12 minutes.

Serve and enjoy.

Nutrition:

Calories 156, Fat 8.4g, Carbohydrates 18.9g, Sugar 11.5g, Protein 1.5g, Cholesterol 55mg.

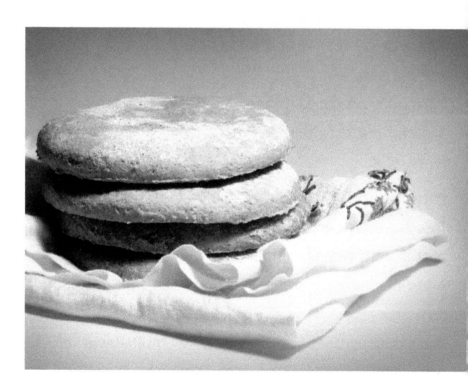

Sweet Potato Chips

Preparation Time: 10 minutes | Cooking Time: 20 minutes | Servings: 2

Ingredients:

1 medium sweet potato, sliced thinly

1/2 tsp ground cinnamon

2 tbsp olive oil

Pepper

Salt

Directions:

Soak sweet potato slices in cold water for 30 minutes. Drain well and pat dry.

Toss sweet potato slices with cinnamon, oil, pepper, and salt.

Place the dehydrating tray in a multi-level air fryer basket and place basket in the Pressure Pot.

Arrange sweet potato slices on a dehydrating tray.

Seal pot with air fryer lid and select air fry mode then set the temperature to 390° F and timer for 20 minutes. Turn halfway through.

Serve and enjoy.

Nutrition:

Calories 173, Fat 14.1g, Carbohydrates 12.3g, Sugar 3.7g, Protein 1.2g, Cholesterol 0mg.

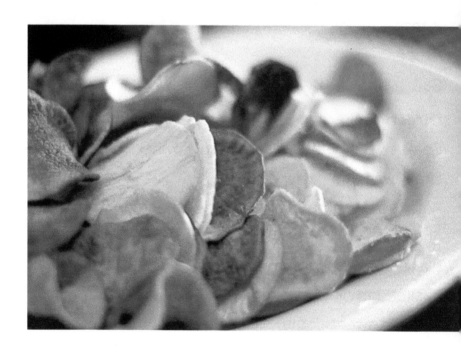

Roasted Baby Potatoes

Preparation Time: 10 minutes | Cooking Time: 20 minutes | Servings: 2

Ingredients:

1/2 lb baby potatoes, clean and cut in half

1/8 tsp thyme

1/4 tsp dried oregano

1/4 tsp dried basil

1/2 tbsp olive oil

Pepper

Salt

Directions:

In a large bowl, toss potatoes with the remaining ingredients.

Spray Pressure Pot multi-level air fryer basket with cooking spray.

Add potatoes into the air fryer basket and place basket into the Pressure Pot.

Seal pot with air fryer lid and select air fry mode then set the temperature to 400° F and timer for 20 minutes. Stir halfway through.

Serve and enjoy.

Nutrition:

Calories 97, Fat 3.6g, Carbohydrates 14.3g, Sugar 0g, Protein 3g, Cholesterol 0mg.

Spicy Chicken Wings

Preparation Time: 10 minutes | Cooking Time: 20 minutes | Servings: 2

Ingredients:

6 chicken wings

1 tbsp olive oil

1 tsp paprika

Pepper

Salt

Directions:

In a bowl, toss chicken wings, paprika, olive oil, pepper, and salt. Cover and place in the refrigerator for 1 hour.

Spray Pressure Pot multi-level air fryer basket with cooking spray.

Add marinated chicken wings into the air fryer basket and place basket into the Pressure Pot.

Seal pot with air fryer lid and select air fry mode then set the temperature to 390° F and timer for 20 minutes. Turn halfway through.

Serve and enjoy.

Nutrition:

Calories 238, Fat 14g, Carbohydrates 0.6g, Sugar 0.1g, Protein 26.8g, Cholesterol 82mg.

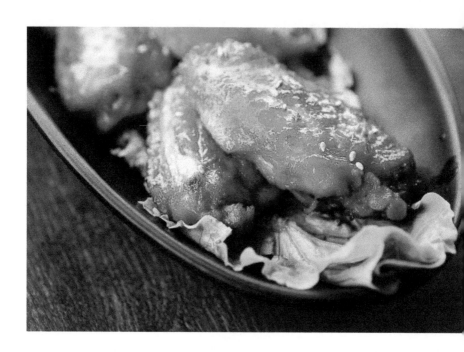

Dry Rub Wings

Preparation Time: 10 minutes | Cooking Time: 14 minutes | Servings: 2

Ingredients:

8 chicken wings

1/2 tsp chili powder

1/2 tsp garlic powder

1/4 tsp pepper

1/4 tsp salt

Directions:

In a bowl, mix chili powder, garlic powder, pepper, and salt.

Add chicken wings to the bowl and toss well.

Spray Pressure Pot multi-level air fryer basket with cooking spray.

Add chicken wings into the air fryer basket and place basket into the Pressure Pot.

Seal pot with air fryer lid and select air fry mode then set the temperature to 350° F and timer for 14 minutes.

Turn halfway through.

Serve and enjoy.

Nutrition:

Calories 242, Fat 9.4g, Carbohydrates 1g, Sugar 0.2g Protein 36.3g, Cholesterol 111mg.

Lightning Source UK Ltd.
Milton Keynes UK
UKHW020807180621
385732UK00001B/94